The Lady's Companion For

First Aid

Treated Naturally

Mark Gilberd
Homoeopath. Medical Herbalist and Iridologist

Contents

Foreword

This book does not replace your First Aid manual but complements its use and allows you to take the best from both worlds. The main purposes of this book is to empower you and give you options that previously you had not, as well as to speed up the healing processes and help relieve pain, stress and trauma. Modern medicine seems to concentrate more on antiseptics and sterile environments especially for wound care but not much on the actual healing processes of the wound especially when you consider that some antiseptics can burn the wound while doing its germ killing. Anyone like me who has had straight iodine poured into deep puncture wounds can vouch for that.

In this booklet we will concentrate on the healing and closing of wounds along with the knitting together of bones with remedies that concentrate on healing as well as having germicide and antibacterial properties. A lot of the emphasis is on finding the cause or causes of the problem and removing them as prevention is the best way to go for good health and a long life. This book gives you the options of Herbal or Homoeopathic remedies or of using them together.

Most of the Remedies mentioned can be acquired fairly easily and locally with the exception being the tinctures and the Homoeopathics but this will vary from country to country.

Natural First Aid

Abscesses - Boils and Carbuncles

These are typically caused by a bacterial infection usually starting in a hair follicle. The first stage is characterized by a painful red swelling after which pus begins to form; this will usually discharge itself in a few days. Do not squeeze as this usually causes internal damage and a spread of the wound and infection. Lots of boils or recurring boils need professional help so as to remove the cause. Diabetes is a condition that causes boils.

Herbal Treatment

The easiest and fasted method would be to use Tea Tree Oil as this tends to draw out infections and bring them to a head. Start as soon as possible, the earlier the better and apply frequently. Use more diluted if using frequently especially if you have sensitive skin. Hot poultices are very effective at drawing the core out of boils so here we shall use a hot poultice of Slippery Elm (half a tea spoon full) with about 4 drops of Castor Oil which is also good at drawing out unwanted matter and mix this with a bit of boiling water to form a hot paste. Alternative poultices are Linseed or Fenugreek, these need to be ground and boiled first before being applied. Apply to the area and leave on for 20 minutes and repeat several times till suppuration occurs.

After suppuration you can mix together a bit of Calendula and Comfrey creams and apply them to the area. These two herbs working together will speed up the healing time, disinfect and reduce or prevent scaring.

For internal treatment think of the herbs Echinacea and Burdock as these are both blood cleansers that will start to work on the causes of the problem and help to prevent more.

Homoeopathic Treatment

A boil is an infected, reddened, swollen area of the skin usually in a hair follicle or some other pit in the skin. Boils can be very painful while they develop until they come to a head and burst.

Arnica 6C - For crops of boils with a bluish area around them.

Tarantula Cubenis 6C - For painful hard feeling boils that develop rapidly after a slow start especially on the back of the neck or on boils where the skin turns red blue or purple. Give this remedy 3 or 4 times daily along with a Hypericum Lotion compress taped over the area.

Acne

This seems to be a mixture of many factors with a main one being sebum which is the oil produced in the hair follicles which increases production due to the increased hormones in puberty and premenstrual. If chronic seek professional help.

Herbal Treatment

1. Make a face mask of slippery elm as this draws out the impurities and opens the pores.

2. Calendula lotion in a 1 to 20 mix helps to regulate the skins production of oil as well as being disinfecting and healing. You can use the Comfrey cream as well to prevent scaring if needed.

Another Effective Method

1. Tea Tree oil dabbed on effected area frequently especially after you have touched it. Tea Tree tends to draw out the infection and bring it to a head. Use in a weak dilution. Some people with sensitive skin may find the oil to strong.

2. Take the Tissue Salts Calc Sulph and Kali Mur (chemist or health shop will have it) Follow directions on the label.

Bites and Stings

I will cover here just bites from pets and bee and wasp stings. Snakes spiders and jellyfish stings require prompt medical attention. With snake and spider bites apply a pressure bandage to the area and keep the limb still and transport to hospital or better still ring a Ambulance. (You can give rescue remedy).

Animal bites can be treated the same as wounds as they are usually a mixture of puncture, bruising and maybe scratches, treat shock with rescue remedy especially in children. With wounds from animals you should always get a tetanus shot or a booster and always treat with lots of Calendula Lotion so as to prevent infection which is common after animal bites especially from cats. If there is a lot of pain add Hypericum to the lotion.

Herbal Treatment

For insect bites and stings Rescue Remedy taken internally and applied to the sting can bring relief especially in children. Witch hazel cream is good for insect bites and stings.

Wasp stings and Ant bites - apply vinegar or lemon juice

Bee stings - Dab on bicarbonate of soda mixed with water. This can also bring relief to sand fly and sometimes mosquito bites as well. Baking Soda works in two ways, firstly it buffers the acid and then the sodium part draws the poison out. On all stings ice can reduce pain and swelling. Aloe vera may sometimes help.

Homoeopathic Treatment

Can be painful in varying degrees; always follow the normal first aid procedures especially from bites from venomous creatures. After a bite or a sting from a animal or insect take one dose of **Ledum 6C** immediately. If you get no relief try one of the following.

Apis 6C - If the injury swells, burns, stings and looks very red, angry and puffy with swelling, worse for warmth , better for cold applications. This remedy is made from the bee and should always be considered for bee stings.

Arnica 6C - Shock, bruising like pain, soreness and does not want area touched.

Cantharis 6C - Violent burning and smarting pain, blisters may develop.

Staphysagria 6C - Large bites that itch violently with smarting, stinging pain.

Bruises

Arnica is the main remedy that is used for bruising mainly as a lotion or a cream but it must not be used where the skin is broken. If used on broken skin it will cause a bad reaction. Arnica is good for the bruised like pain in limbs and joints which have been over used or sprained as well as your everyday type of bruises. For accidents where you hit your finger with the hammer especially when the fingernail is involved put your finger under the cold water tap and leave it there till it nearly feels numb with the cold, this if done fast enough can save you from a bruised nail and a lot of pain.

Herbal Treatment

For bruises where there are open wounds such as cuts and grazes use Witch hazel and Calendula together in a lotion and later you could mix the creams together and apply as healing resumes. For your normal everyday bruises rub Arnica cream gently on the area. If a nerve rich area such as the elbow is bruised add Hypericum to the lotion.

For internal treatment take a Vitamin C powder with

hesperidin, rutin and the bioflavonoids as this will help to repair the damaged capillaries. If you bruise easily consider taking this powder regularly as you may be deficient.

Homoeopathic Treatment

The black and blue appearance of a bruise are caused from blood vessels that have ruptured under the skin as a result of trauma, as the blood from the broken vessels is slowly absorbed the color becomes paler then red or yellow.

Arnica 6C - For bruised soft tissues, muscles and connective tissue. Rapidly aids in the absorption of effused blood. The swelling which usually accompany bruising reduces fairly quickly but if there is little reaction use Ledum 6C. Arnica cream can be used on the external area of the wound.

Caution - Arnica lotion or cream must not be used on or near broken skin only use Calendula or Hypericm cream on wounds.

Ledum 6C - Helps in blood reabsorbing, may be needed if swelling remains after taking Arnica. Affected parts are cold and worse for warmth.

Hypericum 6C - For bruised nerves, use where there is sharp shooting pains in punctured or penetrating wounds, for bruises of nerve rich areas such as the fingers, tail bone, lips and nose. Hypercal cream can be applied to the site externally.

Ruta 6C - Bruises of the bone or the bone covering the periosteum, good for shin bone injuries.

Note - Hypercal cream can be used externally on bruises where the skin is broken as Arnica cream or lotion cannot be used on broken skin.

Bleeding

The main rule for bleeding is to apply pressure to the wound so as to stop the bleeding. For a normal type of slow blood flow from a wound that is persistent Calendula tincture applied with pressure on a pad will usually stop the bleeding, make sure you hold it there for a few minutes.

For the more scary type of bleeding Witch hazel tincture can be used on a pad and applied with pressure to the wound as this herb is much more astringent then Calendula, this extra astringency should cause the ends of the blood vessels to spasm and close off the injured vessels.

Herbal Treatment

Calendula for slow bleeding wounds.

Witch hazel for the fast bleeding wounds.

I would be inclined here to mix the tincture half water half tincture as this would still work and be less painful as the alcohol in the tincture is much more reduced.

See also Cuts and Wounds and consider using Hypercal (Hypericum and Calendula mixed together)

Homoeopathic Treatment

Use normal first aid procedures, apply pressure to the wound, if there is a lot of blood loss seek medical help and be on the lookout for shock.

Arnica 6C - For bleeding after injury, helps with the shock and bruising.

Bone Injuries and Fractures

The main remedy here is Comfrey or to use its old fashioned name knitbone. This is good to use on the injured area when the cast is removed as it will help to strengthen the mend. For areas that cannot have casts on or for fine fractures Comfrey is ideal and will speed up the healing process.

Comfrey has a chemical in it that speeds up cell division it is also astringent and mucilage which gives it soothing and protecting qualities and has been used for hundreds of years in the healing of bones and wounds. Some people grow this herb and then turn it into liquid manure as it is one of the most mineral rich herbs around.

Herbal Treatment

Apply cream to affected area regularly, if you grow comfrey in your garden you can make a poultice out of the leaves and apply it to the affected area.

Homoeopathic Treatment

Follow normal first aid procedures, if the bone is obviously broken it is best to call a ambulance. If you do have to move the patient make sure the injured limb is supported or a sharp piece of bone may cut an internal artery. Most bone injuries need x-rays to determine the extent of the damage.

Arnica 6C - Can be given straight away for the shock and will help ease the pain from the bruising and swelling.

Ledum 6C - Take after Arnica 4 hourly or 3 times a day to assist in the absorption of the extravasation of blood after a fracture so as to reduce the swelling which may take up to 3 to 4 days. (Helps to absorb the internal bleeding after a fracture)

After the bones have been set properly use these two remedies

Calc Phos 6X - Helps in nutrition especially of the bones and promotes the knitting together of the bones. Helps fractures heal much faster. Can be used in alternation with Symphytum 6C.

Symphytum 6C - More commonly known as Comfrey or knitbone or bone set. The name says it all. Promotes fast healing of bones, use with Calc Phos 6X. Take both 3 times daily till recovered.

Burns

The usual rule is to place the burnt area under cold water as soon as possible. I usually leave it under there till it's nearly numb from the cold. The point to remember here is that when you take let's say your hand away from whatever burnt it the heat from the burn is still traveling inward and will continue to do so for about 15 seconds so this is why you must get to the cold water fast so you can reduce the severity and the depth of the burn. For minor burns and scolds Aloe Vera gel straight from the plants leaf can give quick relief and speed up the healing. In Herbal Medicine we use astringents for burns (with the exception being for burns that cover a very large area) as the tannins in the herbs will seal and protect the burned surface. Tannins also have a antibacterial action so this should help in the prevention of infections. Deep burns always require prompt medical attention.

Herbal Treatment

Aloe Vera - apply to burn straight from the plant.

Witch Hazel - Use as a lotion at about 1 to 20 strength and apply to the burn, this herb is a strong astringent and should seal and protect the surface.

Hypericum - This can be added to the above lotion as it has some similar actions but for burns we are mainly using it to reduce the pain.

Once the healing has begun you can continue applying aloe vera especially if there is still pain. Another good herb for around the edges of the burn as it heals is Calendula Cream.

Homoeopathic Treatment

On first degree burns the skin becomes red only. 2nd degree the burn begins to destroy living tissue, blisters develop, 3rd degree the burns are deep and involve all layers of the skin, these are life threatening depending on the size of the area mainly through the loss of fluids and the risk of infections.

Urtica Urens 6C - For first degree burns take as

needed internally for the pain with Hypericum lotion used externally.

Causticum 6C - For 2nd degree burns take as needed for the pain with Hypericum lotion used externally on the burn and Calendula cream on the edges.

Cantharis 6C - For 3rd degree burns taken as needed. This time wait for the healing to begin before using Hypericum and Calendula.

Hypericum Tincture - To be used as a lotion 20 drops of tincture to 1 cup of water.

Calendula Cream - Use this on the edges of the burn.

Cuts and Wounds

The first consideration is to stop the bleeding, rule out any deeper internal damage and clean and disinfect the wound. To stop the bleeding refer to bleeding section. Calendula is one of the main lotions used for cleaning wounds as it is gentle, soothing, astringent, healing and anti-microbial so it kills the germs as well. Calendula has a tendency of sometimes welding the skin together (handy for closing knife cuts) this is more noticeable on wounds with clean cut edges. Because of this tendency it is very important to make sure that all wounds are very clean and no dirt remains inside. Now we will introduce you to Hypericum (St Johns Wort) I use Hypericum lotion on wounds that are in very nerve rich areas, a good example is crush injuries to the finger as we all know how painful and sensitive a wound is to this area. As well as being used for nerve damage Hypericm is also astringent so it will help in stopping the bleeding and its anti-inflammatory action should help to reduce the swelling. I usually get a separate bottle and fill it up with half Hypericum and half Calendula tincture and call this bottle Hypercal. I use this bottle for making my lotions for wounds on nervy areas. Consider also that these are both astringents so our power to stop bleeding has been increased.

Tea Tree Oil is good for small wounds and has a strong antibacterial action but can sometimes hurt in open wounds. The oil is good where there is infection as it draws pus to a head. And now for something completely different. If you have a clean cut wound fairly deep but on the border line of getting stitches and have managed to stop the bleeding here's a way of putting a kind of skin graft on it which will hold the wound shut while you decide what to do. Break and empty an egg. On the inside of the egg shell you will see a plastic like skin, peel this off and lay across the wound wet side down. The skin is also meant to have an antibiotic action which protects the egg. If you are going to try to get away without stitches try to immobilize the area for a couple of days so you don't accidentally rip the wound open again and use plenty of Calendula to close the wound.

Herbal Treatment

1. Deal with bleeding and clean wound under running tap water if possible.

2. Do the final cleaning with Calendula or Hypercal lotion mixed 1 to 20 parts water.

3. Cover and protect the wound if you think it is necessary.

4. When wound is dry and healing (if weeping use Hypercal lotion) you can use Calendula cream with maybe Comfrey cream as well for scar prevention or if the wound is healing slowly. You can also medicate a little bit of Calendula cream with Hypericum to make a Hypercal cream for a healing wound giving off nervy pain.

Homoeopathic Treatment

Use normal first aid techniques, control bleeding etc. When you have everything under control and are ready to see to the wound the best way to start is usually to clean the area with water running from a tap washing everything away from the wound. Calendula lotion is our main treatment for wounds as it is gentle, encourages healing, stops bleeding and no germs can survive in its presence. Use plenty of lotion on the wound and in deep ones let it get into all the cavities. Calendula can make wounds close up very fast especially if they have clean sharp edges so great care must be taken to ensure the wound is clean. Calendula is a great help to old and infected wounds and can usually turn the condition around in a few days. (See Tea Tree oil)

Hypericum is the next most well used lotion, its main calling is for wounds of the very nervy parts of the body such as the fingers, tail bone, lips or for any part that really hurts and is nervy. One of the leading symptoms for Hypericum is shooting pains along the nerve pathways from the injured area. Hypericum is good for infections and septic conditions in nervy areas and I would use it with Calendula for any infection in a wound especially deep wounds. In the past Hypericum was used to prevent Tetanus in deep puncture wounds especially from rusty metal objects. Remember infections are trying to get the rubbish out of the body so when they begin to discharge do not try to stop the discharge let the body get rid of its rubbish.

Hypercal - Which is a half and half mixture of Hypericum and Calendula tinctures, you can use this to make lotions when you want the effects of both Calendula and Hypericum together. A example would be an infected crushed finger.

Creams - Calendula and Hypericum creams can be used when the healing begins and are applied for the same reasons as the lotions but always remember the lotion gets in better. Creams are more for the latter stages of healing.

Arnica 6C - For shock, bruised sore pain of the wound, doesn't like effected area being touched.

Ledum 6C - Used for puncture wounds, prevents tetanus.

Puncture Wounds

Splinters and accidents from stepping on pins, rusty nails, barbed wire or from tools can be dealt with very effectively with homoeopathic remedies.

Arnica 6C - Can help bring splinters to the surface and deal with any shock.

Hypericum 6C - Intense pain shoots up from injured parts especially from those in nerve rich areas, if given immediately with the lotion it can prevent tetanus from developing but it is always best to get a booster shot.

Ledum 6C - This remedy also helps to prevent tetanus and can be used for the same injuries as Hypericum but with Ledum the part feels cold and is relieved by cold, there is puffiness and a pale mottled appearance.

Hypercal Lotion - Externally use a lotion of Hypercal making sure plenty gets inside the wound.

After Surgery

Homoeopathic remedies used before and immediately after surgery will speed up the healing process considerably. Not only does this get you over the problem sooner but it also helps in the prevention of post-operative complications such as hemorrhage, inflammation, and infection. Will also help with the internal healing and bruising.

Aconite 6C - Great fear and anguish with restlessness. Possible fear of death, great suddenness of symptoms. This is a good one to think of before surgery.

Arnica 6C - Bruised sore pain with fear of being touched. Take this immediately before and straight after a operation.

Bellis Perennis 6C - Follows after and is similar to Arnica but is used for the deeper internal bruising while Arnica is more external. Good for trauma and wounds of the pelvic and abdominal organs.

Hypericum 6C - For damage to tissue rich in nerves or the nerves themselves, pains shoot along nerve pathways.

Staphysagria 6C - Stinging, cutting, smarting pains after surgery, good for knife cut like wounds. This remedy has strong mental symptoms of Feels as if the body has been invaded, or a sense of humiliation after a physical exam, resentment and anger to hospital staff may be present.

Calendula Lotion - This is our main lotion and cream used for wounds. Apply the lotion to the wound and surrounding area as Calendula is very soothing and healing. Latter when the wound is healing Calendula cream can be used.

Hypercal Lotion - Is a mixture of Calendula and Hypericum tinctures that are used as a lotion. The Calendula is used for its healing, anti-microbial, anti-hemorrhagic and soothing properties while the Hypericum is used for the nervy type of pain from the wounds in nerve rich areas.

The lotion is mixed at a strength of 1 to 20 parts water or stronger if needed.

Diarrhea

Diarrhea is a natural bodily process that is used to rid the body of toxins, infections or irritants of any kind so unless it continues for too long it should not be suppressed. Lots of fluids should be taken and in some cases it may be wise to stay off food for 24 hours. Always try to find the cause; it may be from stress, viruses, bacterial infection or maybe a food allergy.

Herbal Treatment

Chamomile tea can be given if the symptoms match as this is calming, soothing, and antispasmodic and will help to heal the irritation and if you put a pinch of ginger in the tea this would also help to relieve nausea if it is present. Always think of Chamomile if nerves or worry are the cause. Slippery elm powder in water also soothes the irritation and relieves the diarrhea as well as being nourishing. Agrimony is our specific for diarrhea especially in children. Witch Hazel due to it astringency helps in the control of diarrhea and may help in reducing dysentery but like agrimony it is better to give in tea form as this allows maximum contact with the intestines as it travel through so it can medicate a far wider area.

The aim of treatment is to help the body rid itself of the toxins rather than suppressing the problem. Garlic oil capsules may be taken if you are reasonably sure that the problem is caused from a virus or bacterial infection. (See herb list at back for more information on this). If the problem continues longer than it should seek medical advice.

Dysentery

Dysentery is when the above problem continues and there is colicky like pains with maybe wind and gurgling with the motions becoming more water like. Herbal treatment of this condition mainly concentrates on the actions of the astringent herbs which contract the tissue and slow down the motions, the main one to think of here is Agrimony with maybe Witch Hazel added so as to increase the astringency. To the astringents you can add herbs like Peppermint, Ginger and Chamomile which will help with the tummy cramps, colic, wind and pain. Slippery Elm is a very gentle astringent and also provides the body with nutrition and if you add a bit of unprocessed honey to it your giving extra energy and an antibacterial action as well. When dealing with the intestines always use the remedies in tea form as tis allows the tea to spread through a large area medicating as it goes.

Emergency Rehydration Fluid
1 litre of boiled water
2 tea spoonful's of salt
2 tablespoons of sugar
Mix together and sip regularly throughout the day

Ear Ache

Try to find the cause, is it an acute infection, tooth ache, from sinus problems etc. Recurring ear infections need professional help so as to build up the immune system to cope. Seek medical help if the pain is excessive or there is pain in the mastoid bone (behind the ear) or any discharge.

The juice of garlic or alternatively onion in olive oil warmed to body temperature but no more can be put in the ear but only if the drum is not perforated. If the drum is perforated they will be in great pain and there may be a discharge. To get the juice from a onion slice it thinly into circles and lay flat in a saucer and sprinkle a bit of sugar on it then put another layer of onion more sugar etc and keep building it up. When finished leave for at least a hour and the sugar will draw out the juice.

Herbal Treatment

Garlic or onion juice in olive oil warmed to body temperature.

Eczema and Dermatitis

Is an irritating skin inflammation that may be due to a allergy caused by certain foods or from repeated contact to certain chemicals (dermatitis) or just inherited. This condition can be made worse from stress. This is more of a problem needing professional help except for contact dermatitis which can be cured by removing the cause or to a certain degree through the use of a barrier cream.

Weeping eczema requires a wet dressing of Chamomile (anti-inflammatory) and Witch hazel (astringent) which should start to dry the area out. Once the weeping has stopped you can use Calendula and Comfrey creams which will start healing and give some relief. Chickweed lotion can be used as a wet dressing as well, the leading symptoms for this is itching and irritation with the main emphasis on itching. You can if you want medicate some cream with a few drops of Chickweed tincture and can use this cream to relieve any itching that may happen when healing is in progress. A good mix for this cream would be Calendula.

Herbal Treatment

For weeping eczema Chamomile tea used as a lotion mixed with Witch hazel lotion made at 1 to 10 parts water. This mixed lotion is applied as a wet bandage to the area (moisten bandage frequently) or you can wet a pad with the lotion and bandage that to the area till weeping has stopped.

Replace Chamomile with Chickweed lotion if symptoms are very itchy with irritation. For dry eczema Comfrey and Calendula cream used together will speed up the healing if itching is a problem you can medicate some Calendula cream with a few drops of Chickweed tincture.

Eye Problems

See also conjunctivitis. Eyebright as you can guess is the main herb for the eye and is used for most eye problems and even for just sore or strained eyes it can be soothing. For a little splinter in the eye or a hard to remove foreign body a few drops of Castor oil can be used for its drawing power as it has a good reputation for removing embedded objects and it will sooth the irritation at the same time. If the eye is irritated and you have suspicion there is something in put a few drops of Castor oil in before you go to sleep and leave overnight and the problem will usually be gone by the morning.

Herbal Treatment

Eyebright lotion at 1 to 20 parts water in a eyebath (always try in a very diluted form first, 2 drops to a eyebath) for sore red eyes or better still as a compress especially with hay fever symptoms.

Castor oil 2 or 3 drops into the eye to draw out foreign bodies and relieve irritation. Best left overnight.

Conjunctivitis

The conjunctiva is a delicate membrane which covers the whites of the eyes. This may become inflamed due to irritation, infection or allergic reaction. Try to avoid touching and rubbing the eye as this usually irritates it more and if it is an infection there is a chance that it may spread to the other eye. The herbs to use here are Calendula and Eyebright used as lotions in the strength of 1 to 20 parts water. Eyebright is a very astringent herb so you would use it if the eye was very watery and inflamed while Calendula is soothing and anti-infective. If the eye was watery and infected you could mix both the herbs together for a more effective treatment.

Herbal Treatment

Calendula lotion 1 to 20 in a eyebath (healing and soothing).

Eyebright Lotion 1 to 20 in a eyebath (astringents will help in stopping watering and help with the inflammation).

Homoeopathic Treatment

Here I will cover mainly blows to the eyes and the simple removal of foreign objects and will also give you one of the main eye remedies. For a blow to the eye you can give Arnica 6C or Aconite 6C which has been called the Arnica of the eye, a leading symptom for Aconite 6C is if the eye feels gritty or as if something is in the eye. If pain is felt in the eyeball give Symphytum 6C.

Arnica 6C is more suited for a black eye (see bruising).

After removal of a foreign object from the eye Aconite 6C can be given and if the eye is still sensitive and sore an eye bath of water with 2 drops of Euphrasia (Eye Bright) tincture can be tried.

Arnica 6C - For shock and bruising.

Acconite 6C - For the suddenness of the condition and shock, pain feels like a piece of grit in the eye, eye looks red and inflamed.

Euphrasia Lotion - Conjunctivitis after injury, eyes are hot, burning and watering, soreness, eye strain. 2 drops of tincture into a eye bath full of water gives relief to sore and wind burnt eyes. You can also use Euphrasia 6C internally at the same time.

Symphytum 6C - for blows to the eyeball itself, blunt injury trauma such as a tennis or squash ball.

Gastritis and Gastroenteritis

Gastritis or inflammation of the stomach can often be from overindulgence or upsetting foods and can lead to nausea, vomiting, diarrhea and heartburn. Symptoms are usually short lived. Gastroenteritis is usually more serious it can have the above symptoms with abdominal cramps added. In children the commonest cause is a virus but it can be caused by bacteria from contaminated food. This can be serous in children and small babies since the constant vomiting and diarrhea can lead to dehydration. Always consider a fast for 24 hours so the system has a chance to recover.

Peppermint or Chamomile infusion every hour for the first day, you could even take them alternately if you think the symptoms call for this. After this one cup 3 or 4 times daily for a week before breakfast, between meals and before bed. These infusions should bring relief to pain, fever and spasms in the digestive tract. Slippery elm powder taken with a lot of water will soothe, help heal and reduce irritation and over active peristalsis. A little bit of Cardamom could be put in the infusions and this might help with any vomiting and help to settle the stomach. In digestive problems always use the tea form (infusion) of the herb for treatment as this allows a far greater volume area to be medicated.

Herbal Treatment

Agrimony -Iinflammation, mucous colitis, indigestion, appendicitis and diarrhea.

Chamomile tea - anti-inflammatory, anti-spasmodic, carminative and pain killer.

Peppermint tea - anti spasmodic, carminative, diaphoretic, anti-emetic (prevents vomiting), anti-septic, pain killing.

Cardamom - Carminative, stomach tonic, digestive tonic.

Slippery elm powder in water - soothing, astringent, nutritive.

For gastroenteritis stop all foods and avoid milk and milk based products for a least 24 hours. Refer to other sections for vomiting, nausea and diarrhea.

Hay Fever

This is more a deep seated type of problem that needs Professional help. Before the season begins start preparing the body, consider a non-mucous forming diet, start taking Vit C daily for it is a natural anti histamine and one of the main anti-oxidants for the lungs. Start taking Garlic daily as this will start clearing out the system with its anti-bacterial and anti-viral actions along with its high content of sulphur. Before the season and throughout the season take the formula below about 3 times a day.

Elder Flowers 2 parts

Chamomile 1 part

Eyebright 1 Part

Golden Seal 1 part

For relief of the eyes you can try a Euphraisa eye bath. Add 2 drops of tincture to the water in the eye bath and mix well. (See eye problems)

Homoeopathic Treatment

Hay fever is a allergic condition affecting the mucous membranes of the eyes, nose and air passages in people who are sensitive to pollens and grasses. Typical symptoms are running nose or eyes with a stuffed up sensation with may be itching of the eyes, nose or throat.

Allium Cepa 6C - Frequent sneezing with heavy burning nasal discharge and bland watery discharge from the eyes. The smell of flowers aggravates.

Euphrasia 6C - Red, burning, itching, watering eyes, water from the eyes burns the skin while the nasal discharge is bland. (Opposite to Allium Cepa).

Hemorrhoids or Piles

Hemorrhoids are a painful condition that really needs Professional help so as to remove the cause. For self-help treatment Witch hazel, Calendula and Hypericum creams can be used with Witch hazel being the main remedy as its strong astringency will stop any bleeding and help reduce the size of the pile a lot faster. If you have a feeling this condition is coming on attack the area straight away with Witch hazel cream and keep at it, if you are prone to piles you will find that this is a good and effective treatment that may sometimes prevent the condition from occurring. If you keep the cream in the fridge you will find that it is more relieving.

Herbal Treatment

Witch hazel cream - Apply immediately even on suspicion.
Calendula cream - Healing, soothing and antiseptic.
Hypericum cream - Will help with itching and pain. Also consider Chickweed for the itching.
All of the above can be used in lotion form to clean the area.

Indigestion

Indigestion or dyspepsia can have many symptoms varying from heart burn to bloating with maybe nausea and abdominal discomfort somewhere in the middle. There can be many causes some of which are not chewing food properly, eating too fast, too much rich or fatty foods, or if you are finding that this is getting to be a common problem the cause may be from low levels of stomach acid, stress or poor pancreas or liver function so it would be wise to seek professional help. You can mix and make your individual formula from the herbs below or just use one at a time.

Herbal Treatment

Slippery elm for heart burn or acidy symptoms mix with water.

Agrimony -Inflammation, mucous colitis, indigestion, appendicitis and diarrhea.

Licorice is a strong demulcent and can sooth areas hurt from excess acid.

Ginger capsules or in a mixed tea for flatulence, dyspepsia, colic and nausea.

Peppermint tea stimulates bile and digestive juices, flatulence, nausea.

Chamomile tea for indigestion, inflammations and colic and cramping like sensations.

Cardamom added to any of these will help.

In digestive problems always use the tea form (infusion) of the herb for treatment as this allows a far greater volume area to be medicated.

Itching

Itching can have many different causes some are from fungal infections, hemorrhoids, intestinal worms (itchy anus), liver problems, allergies, bites, stings etc.

Treating the cause should relieve the problem but for temporary relief for the skin you could try a baking powder paste (good for sand flies etc) or some Chickweed cream or lotion.

Herbal Treatment

Chickweed cream or lotion - Apply to itchy areas.

Baking powder - Mix with water to make a paste and apply to itchy area. Usually draws out the toxin causing the itch and if the toxin is acid it will alkalize it.

Motion Sickness

This can be car sickness, air sickness and sea sickness the remedy to take here is ginger.

Herbal Treatment

Ginger - Take a few capsules just before the trip.

Peppermint.-. Take as a tea or you can buy peppermint oil capsules from a chemist.

Nose Bleed

The usual rule for this is to lean your head right back and pinch the top of your nose and stay this way till the bleeding is stopped. If you are still having problems after that you can get a small piece of cotton wool and soak it in a strong lotion of witch hazel and insert it in the nose (make sure it is a long piece so you can get it out easily) and pinch your nose gently, the idea is for the lotion to make contact with the wound and the astringency of the lotion should close the blood vessels.

Herbal Treatment

Witch hazel lotion at about 4 to 10 parts water strength applied as described above.

Nausea

Try to find the cause, common ones are digestive upsets, nerves, motion, migraines, liver problems and pregnancy. The main herbs to use here are chamomile, peppermint and ginger.

Refer to the herbal at the back and try to match your symptoms to the herbs you may have to mix a few herbs together to cover everything or maybe even all three.

Herbal Treatment

Chamomile tea - Colic, cramps, nervy.

Peppermint tea - Stimulates bile and digestive juices, good if cause is from food

Ginger tea or capsules - Good for nausea and vomiting and gentle for those who are pregnant.

Cardamom added to any of these will help.

In digestive problems always use the tea form (infusion) of the herb for treatment as this allows a far greater volume area to be medicated.

Ringworm

Ringworm is a fungal infection which usually attacks when the immune system is weakened by stress or exhaustion. Fungi thrive in damp, dark and confined places. If you think your immune system is run down you can take Echinacea, Zinc, and Vitamin C and you might as well take Garlic as this has an anti-fungal action. Externally treatment can be a lotion of Calendula 1 to 5 strength for cleaning the area and around it. Stronger anti fungals may be necessary as this can sometimes be a very stubborn condition to get rid of. Garlic is a stronger anti-fungal and you can use this externally (break open a Garlic oil capsule) and internally at the same time.

Herbal Treatment

Raise immunity if needed refer to influenza for the method.

Calendula lotion 1 to 5 strength on and around the affected area.

Tea tree oil - strong anti-fungal dab on to the affected area neat.

Garlic externally on effected area and latter if problem is not resolving take internally.

Sunburn

A lotion of Witch hazel and Hypericum would help the burn and relieve the pain. If you have a Aloe Vera plant you could rub the gel on the burn. Be sure to rehydrate. Refer to the burns section.

Herbal Treatment

A mixture of Witch hazel and Hypericum lotion 1 to 20 parts water.

Sprains

Severe sprains usually need a supporting bandage and a medical checkup to see if there has been any other damage. A lot of damage and trauma can be prevented if the injured area was put under cold water or ice immediately after the injury the quicker the less the damage. For a bad sprain I would use lots of Arnica cream to start with and at night apply Arnica and Comfrey mixed creams along with a support bandage for the area so as to keep the cream there and also for the extra heat to the area that would create. If you grow Comfrey in your garden then you could put on a Comfrey poultice at night. Ginger is another herb that could be used in a poultice at night. In the past they also used what was known as Hot and Cold Treatment especially for ankles. It works like this put the swollen ankle in a bucket of hot water as hot as they can bear leave for about 5 minutes then put in a bucket of very cold water for 5 minutes, keep repeating the process, this probably works like a mechanical pump eg hot expands cold contracts so you may be pumping the inflammatory swelling out and fresh blood in leading to decongestion and fast healing.

A very fast method of treating strains and sprains is with Glucosamine, Chondroitin and MSM in the powdered form, you should be able to find this at most chemists. Glucosamine is an anti-inflammatory while the chondroitin helps rebuild cartilage and heal joints and attachments. You use this in the powdered form dissolved in water as it is rapidly absorbed by the intestine and enters the blood which takes it to the injury. A lot of athletes and horses use this frequently during the day along with the hot and cold treatment to force heal their injuries so they can compete again as soon as possible. Three times a day is good enough for the rest of us.

Herbal Treatment

Cold water or ice immediately.
Arnica cream (do not apply on open wounds).
Comfrey Cream mixed with Arnica cream overnight.
Ginger poultice overnight.

Homoeopathic Treatment

Joint problems due to twisting, wrenching or over use. A sprain is damaged tendons or ligaments while a strain happens when the connecting tissues around a joint are over stretched. Use your normal first aid procedures and support the joint with supporting bandage and give the appropriate remedies with the first one being Arnica. If there is no sign of improvement in 24 to 36 hours get checked for a fracture.

Arnica 6C - For the shock and bruised sore pains. Arnica cream can also be applied as long as the skin is not broken.

Bellis Perennis 6C - Deeper acting then Arnica, intense soreness of the muscles, where swellings and lumps remain after the injury.

Ledum 6C - Injuries where the swollen part is cold or numb, sometimes looks purple and puffy, feels better for cold applications.

Ruta 6C - If the bones inside or near the joint feel bruised

Splinters

This is here for splinters so deep you can't remove or those really annoying ones that you can feel but can't see. To get these out we will use a poultice. There are two to choose from, the first is a Slippery elm poultice made by adding hot water and turning into a paste and applying to the wound site, cover and secure with a bandage and renew every 2 hours till drawn out.

The other is Castor oil, with this one it is easier to put it on cotton wool and apply it to the wound at night so it can work while you are sleeping.

Herbal Treatment

Slippery elm poultice

Castor oil compress

Shock

All accidents and emergencies cause a certain degree of emotional shock sometimes very noticeable in children. Shock should always be treated along with any other injuries. Signs of shock can be they look pale, cold and sweaty skin, restless, rapid pulse and there may be shallow and fast breathing. Lay them down and get them comfortable keep them warm and calm and reassure them. Loosen tight clothing. Rescue Remedy is a effective remedy for this condition and can be used for any type of shock physical or emotional. Emotionally it will relieve that uptight feeling or apprehension before a certain event. Rescue Remedy is a mixture of five Bach Flower Remedies and has been used since the late 30s so it has been well proved and is easily found in most health shops and chemists.

Herbal Treatment

Rescue Remedy - For physical and emotional shock in any circumstances.

Homoeopathic Treatment

As you would of noticed by now Arnica is our main remedy for shock with Aconite being a very good second remedy if the symptoms match. Don't forget to follow all your normal first aid procedures and keep the patient warm and calm.

Acconite 6C - Severe shock with great fear and restlessness. Fear is so great, person may scream, or say they will die, useful after surgical shock.

Arnica 6C - Reduces shock and hemorrhage and helps relieve the pain.

Notes

Our Two Main Wound Herbs

Calendula

Medicinal Actions - Anti-inflammatory, astringent, vulnerary, anti-fungal, germicide, demulcent.

Part Used - The Flowers

Used For.-. Minor skin problems, cuts, abrasions, rashes, spots, acne, sore nipples Slow healing wounds, skin ulcers and to improve post-operative healing Fungal skin infections such as thrush, athletes foot and ring worm. Used to stop bleeding, heal bruises and sprains, skin ulcers, minor burns and scolds, healing, soothing, anti-microbial. As a douche or bath to treat vaginal thrush, Gargle for sore throat and tonsillitis It can be applied as a lotion, ointment, wash, gargle, compress, poultice, bath and douche as required. . Use as a lotion (1 to 20) to clean wounds, one of our main germicides for wounds and if Hypericum is added to the lotion you may prevent tetanus as well

Caution - Calendula closes wounds rapidly so make sure they are very clean and no foreign bodies remain.

How To Use – For very serious wound bleeding medicate cloth with tincture and apply with pressure to the area till bleeding stops. Use as a Lotion one part tincture to twenty parts water to wash out wounds or medicate affected area, make at 1 to 10 for bleeding or fungal infections. Use a teaspoon of tincture to medicate a small jar of cream then stir rapidly for 5 minutes or less if it mixes in fast, usually they don't. I usually get a cheap Vitamin E cream from one of the big cheap wholesalers and medicate the cream with Calendula. Use Tincture for medicating creams.

History - The common name for Calendula officinalis is Marigold and it is also known as pot or garden marigold or Mary's Gold. The Latin name is derived from the Latin term calends, which became our English word for calendar, and describes its nature to flower in almost every month of the year. The petals were used by the Romans as a substitute for saffron. The flower petals of the calendula or pot marigold, have been used for medicinal purposes since at least the 12th century. Calendula is native to the Mediterranean. Europeans have long used the orange petals of Calendula to color butter and cheese. The use of Marigold as a medicinal plant has been recorded in traditional herbal literature for hundreds of years. Culpepper's Complete Herbal (1653) describes marigolds as 'being so plentiful in every garden, and so well known that they need no description'. Calendula was eaten widely at this time which is where it gets its name, pot marigold i.e. for the cooking pot. Both Culpepper describes its use as a soothing treatment for skin inflammation, swelling, infections, ulcers and varicose veins. It was also found to be beneficial against smallpox and measles to reduce fever and bring out the spots and hence healing (Culpepper, 1653

Herbal Actions of Calendula

Germicide - Calendula is a strong antiseptic, due to it wide variety of chemical constituents, including **carotenoids** which speed up wound healing and strengthens cells. Along with fighting bacteria in topical preparations, Calendula also fights viruses and fungi, particularly those on the skin and nails.

Anti-inflammatory - Where-ever there is skin irritation and redness, an anti-inflammatory action is needed to help the skin recover. With Calendula also being a Germicide it also takes out the cause of the inflammation which is usually infection. Here the **triterpene alcohols** in calendula exert their powerful inflammation reducing effects. They contribute to the plants overall ability to heal wounds such as burns, cuts and grazes as effectively or more effectively than conventional steroidal applications.

Astringent - The most important use of the astringents in First Aid is to stop the bleeding and they do this by causing the arterioles and arteries to spasm at the cut end. Calendula is well known for stopping bleeding especially in the hard to stop areas such as the palms of hands where in the serious cases tinctures can be used on cloth and put in the palm and the patient made to make a fist. Calendulas astringent action. can be used to improve blood vessel tone and tighten up skin cells, thus reducing the occurrence of complaints such as hemorrhoids.(use with Witchazel and Hypericum) Many new mums find themselves looking for a natural way to combat this condition and it is important to do so as there is a risk of developing blood clots. Calendula once again is the medicine of choice as it contains **hydroxycoumarins**, anti-thrombotic agents that can prevent this from happening. The plant also contains **flavonoids** which improve circulation by boosting the health of capillaries.

Demulcent - The soothing properties of Calendula are due to many of its chemical constituents, in particular the **triterpene saponins** and **mucilage**. Both of these substances provide a soft and 'demulcent' healing effect on external skin surfaces. Another significant component of Calendula is the **essential oil** which is used in many skin formulations and is aromatic and soothing to smell. These are all reasons why Calendula is such a great nutritive for the skin and the best choice for the sensitive skin of a baby.

Anti-oxidant - Of the many therapeutic actions of calendula this is the most celebrated and it is due to the presence of **carotenoids, flavonoids** and **phenolic acids**. Carotenoids are an important cellular nutrient, helping skin to heal faster while flavonoids reduce cellular aging and maximize the integrity of cell walls. Phenolic acids are thought to be protective to cells, in particular those in the cardiovascular system.

Hypericum (St Johns Wort)

Medicinal Actions - Anti-inflammatory, astringent, anti-viral, anti-spasmodic, nervine, vulnerary, antibacterial.

Part Used - Aerial parts

Uses – For First Aid we are concentrating on external use only. Used for wounds with pains that shoot along the nerves, in nerve rich areas such as the fingers, lips, tail bone and toes. As a lotion it will speed the healing of wounds and bruises and is used where there is nerve damage and the possibility of tetanus. The main remedy for puncture wounds. Good for, varicose veins especially the painful kind and mild burns. Patients recovering from surgery where the nerves have been damaged often recover faster with Hypericum. For inflamed joints and rheumatic pain, painful abscesses, bad insect stings, damaged nerves from impact injuries, sprains and ulcers. Eases the pain in conditions such as lumbago, sciatica and Shingles where a cream can be used on the sore and the oil applied along the affected nerve path. As a lotion it is commonly mixed with Calendula, Homoeopaths call this lotion Hypercal.

How To Use - Use as a Lotion one part tincture to twenty parts water to wash out wounds or medicate affected area, make at 1 to 10 for painful and dirty wounds. Mix with Calendula in large painful bleeding wounds with a chance of tetanus. Use Tincture for medicating creams.

History

St. John's Wort has enjoyed a reputation as a wound healer since the fifth century BC. Dioscorides, Paul of Aegina, Pliny, and Galen all referred to the plant, which is said to relieve excessive pain, remove the effects of shock, and have a tonic effect on the mind and body. The name St. John probably refers to John the Baptist, whom tradition said was born on the summer solstice. It was claimed that the red spots visible on the underside of some of the herb's leaves symbolized the blood of St. John, who was beheaded by Herod. In **1907 Ellingwood** a famous Herbalist of the time listed the uses as for muscular bruises, deep soreness, painful parts, a sensation of throbbing in the body without fever. Burning pain, or deep soreness of the spine upon pressure, spinal irritation, and circumscribed areas of intense soreness over the spinal cord or ganglia. Concussional shock or injury to the spine, lacerated or punctured wounds in any location, accompanied with great pain. In the times of horse and carriages Homoeopaths were using it on horses to prevent tetanus after injuries to the hoofs mainly from puncture wounds there from nails or similar objects as these wound on the hoof were prone to tetanus. Hypericum has been one of the main Homoeopathic First Aid Remedies for hundreds of years used by itself or mixed with Calendula in a solution called HYPERCAL. After the 1930's it faded from popularity, but was used by the Russians in WW2 as a replacement for morphine in Lotion and Potencies

Hypercal

Hypercal is a 50 50 mixture of Hypericum and Calendula Tinctures. This is a combination of two of the best wound healing herbs mixed together. Calendula is more for dealing with the blood vessels and bleeding along with the rapid closure of the wound so care must be taken to ensure the wound is clean and no foreign bodies are there to be sealed in. Hypericums work is more on the damaged nerves and pain as well as infections in and of the nervous system especially those caused by deep and painful puncture wounds which could harbor tetanus if not properly cleaned and dealt with. By using these two herbs together you are doubling their main actions of anti-inflammatory and astringents with the last action being good for stopping bleeding and also infection. Wounds calling for Hypercal are usually bloody and painful. Works well on long and extensive grazes and cleaning gravel rash and wounds but is mainly called for impact injuries to the lips, fingers or toes. Ideal for closing clean incisions fast and after surgical operations. So the leading symptoms for Hypercal are painful wounds.

Use as a lotion at one part to ten or 1 to 20 depending on your judgment of pain and infection. In emergency bleeding use the tincture as this will spasm the arterioles but be aware that the high alcohol content will cause pain in its raw state. Use Tincture for medicating creams.

First Aid Herbal

Aloe Vera

Actions - External demulcent, healing, soothing,
Use for sunburn, thermal burns, cuts, sores, inflamed skin, eczema, insect bites.
I suggest you buy a couple of these plants and put them in a handy place.
Part Used - The fresh juice from the leaves

Agrimony

Actions – Astringent, cholagogue, tonic, diuretic.
This is the specific for childhood diarrhea. Used for a number of gastrointestinal problems such as inflammation, mucous colitis, indigestion, appendicitis and diarrhea. Acts as a tonic due to it bitter stimulation. Best given in tea form so it can spread along the intestines and do its job. Consider mixing with licorice for extra soothing and anti-inflammatory action or peppermint but mainly to make it taste better.

Arnica

Actions - Anti-inflammatory, vulnerary.
For external use only Homoeopathic preparations can be used internally. For the treatment of shock and pains from accidents, bruises, joint stiffness and wounds, swellings, paralysis, sprains, rheumatic

conditions or where ever there is inflammation on the skin.

Part Used - The flowers

Caution - Do not apply to open wounds or broken skin.

Calendula

Actions - Anti-inflammatory, astringent, vulnerary, anti-fungal.

Used for cuts, grazes, infected sores, fungal infections, any skin inflammations, regulates the oil production of the skin so is good for acne, to stop bleeding, bruises and sprains, skin ulcers, minor burns and scolds, healing, soothing, anti-microbial. Use as a lotion (1 to 20) to clean wounds, one of our main germicides for wounds and if Hypericum is added to the lotion you may prevent tetanus as well.

Part Used - The Flowers

Caution - Calendula closes wounds rapidly so make sure they are very clean and no foreign bodies remain.

Cardamom

Actions - Antispasmodic, carminative, digestive tonic, stomach tonic, appetizer.

Use for anorexia, bloating, bronchitis, celiacs disease, colic, cramps, depression, fatigue, flatulence, indigestion and vomiting, best used mixed with another herb. Cardamom belongs to the ginger family and shares a lot of common properties with ginger and could be looked upon in use as a milder form of ginger.

Part Used - Ripe seed.

Dose - 1 Teaspoon of powder infused. Three cups a day.

Castor Oil

Castor oils main claim to fame is from its purgative action. It is one of the main purgative remedies from the past and still does well today because it is one of the few purgatives that clears the bowels effectively with one dose and has no unpleasant side effects (besides taste) like gripping pain, spasms etc which made it safe to use for pregnant women to use. Castor oil was used in the hospitals of the past for decades. Castor oil is not the cure for constipation but it can be used for relief of this now and again. Castor oil used in a poultice has good drawing out power on foreign objects imbedded in the body such as splinters in the fingers and especially in the eye where it soothes the irritation at the same time.

Chamomile

Actions - Carminative, sedative, anti-spasmodic, anti-inflammatory, analgesic and anti-septic.

Use for indigestion, colic, diarrhea, teething children, anxiety, insomnia, nervous upsets, slowing down hyperactive children, flatulence. It is a famed blood cleanser and pain reducer, reduces tumors (poultice), remedy for female ailments, inflamed gums, use for blood and skin disorders, aches and pains, external and internal inflammations, cleanser and toner of the digestive tract, improves and helps appetite. This herb is also anti-allergy. Good all round tonic for the nervous system.

Part Used - Flowers

Dose - 2 to 4mls 3 times daily of the Tincture, in the tea form 3 to 4 cups per day.

Chickweed

Actions - Healing, anti-inflammatory, astringent, emollient.

One of the main uses of this herb is for itching skin conditions whether from insect bites or eczema like conditions. Has wound healing and demulcent properties.

Part Used - Aerial parts

Dose - Usually given in infusions (tea form) or used as a lotion or cream.

Comfrey

Actions - Demulcent, astringent, healing, expectorant.

Once widely cultivated as a fodder plant, sheep and cows eat it greedily, the impressive wound healing powers of comfrey are partially due to allantoin which stimulates cell proliferation and speeds the healing process inside and out.

Uses - Its old name is knit bone and that describes well what it does. Comfrey also guards against scar tissue from developing incorrectly, all internal hemorrhages, reunion of wound and fractures, internal ulcers, ruptures, pulmonary problems, bronchitis, irritable cough, ulcerative colitis, skin ulcers and varicose veins.

Part Used - Root, rhizome and leaf.

Echinacea

Actions - Immune stimulant, anti-microbial, anti-inflammatory, alterative, healing.

Is a infection fighter active against strep bacteria (abscesses and boils), a blood cleanser, (blood poisons, snake bites, poisonous insects) and a glandular and lymphatic system cleanser. Use it particularly for respiratory infections and for any disease above the waist. This is one of our main immune boosters for the acute diseases.

Uses - All infections, depressed immune function, inflammatory conditions, allergies, effective against both bacteria and viruses.

Part Used - Root

Dose - 1 to 4mls of tincture three times daily, In the tea form 3 to 4 cups per day.

Warning - Do not use continually as you will burn out the immune system use month on month off.

Eye Bright

Actions - Anti-inflammatory, astringent, anti-catarrhal.

As the name says this is one of the main herbs in the treatment of eye problems. The whole plant is also nervine, tonic and astringent. Its use is both internal and external strengthening greatly the eyes nerves when used so. The high potassium and sulphur content of the plant make it also of value in treatment of gastric ailments especially insufficiency of gastric juices. Acts as a internal medicine for the constitutional tendency to eye weakness.

Uses- Best known for its use in the eye where it is helpful in acute or chronic inflammations, stinging and weeping eyes, over sensitivity to light, conjunctivitis, allergies, sinusitis, ulcers and general eye weakness.

Part Used - Dried aerial parts.

Garlic

Actions - Immune stimulant, anti-bacterial, anti-viral, anti-fungal, anti-septic, anti-oxidant, diaphoretic, cholagogue, hypotensive, anti-spasmodic, vermifuge and many more.The plant is rich in volatile oil and sulphur and because of its remarkable penetrating, disinfecting and mucous expelling powers garlic is a valuable basic remedy for the treatment of all ailments in which the cleansing of the blood stream and expulsion of mucous accumulations is required. Garlic is extremely effective in dissolving and cleansing cholesterol from the blood stream, it stimulates the digestive tract, kills worms, parasites and harmful bacteria, normalizes blood pressure, reduces fever, gas and cramps.

Uses- All infections, coughs, colds, flu, bronchitis, all fevers, pulmonary conditions, gastric and skin complaints, rheumatism, all worms, ringworm, ticks and lice. Acts on Bacteria, Viruses and Internal Parasites.

Dose - 1 clove 3 times a day. Garlic oil capsules are good.

Externally - You can use garlic for ring worm and ear ache, to disinfect wounds and sores, parasitical infections.

Ginger

Actions- Carminative, anti-inflammatory, vasodilator, circulatory stimulant, diaphoretic.

Aids in fighting colds, colitis, digestive disorders, wind, increases saliva, is excellent for the circulatory system and helps increase stamina.

Uses- Indigestion, nausea, feverish conditions especially when chills are present, travel sickness especially sea sickness, dyspepsia, colic, flatulence.

Part Used - Root

Dose - Weak tincture 1.5 to 3mls 3 times daily. Can be found in tablets. Teas may also be made.

Caution - Dont use large doses on an empty

stomach..

Hypericum (St Johns Wort)

Actions - Anti-inflammatory, astringent, anti-viral, anti-spasmodic, nervine, vulnerary, antibacterial.

Uses - Taken internally has a sedative and pain reducing effect, neuralgic pain, anxiety, tension, rheumatic pain, sciatica, for pains that shoot along the nerves, as a lotion it will speed the healing of wounds and bruises and is used where there is damage to the nerve rich areas, varicose veins and mild burns. Good for inflamed joints and rheumatic pain. Recently the herb has become popular to use as a antidepressant especially for cases of anxiety. Use as a lotion on wounds especially in the nerve rich areas such as the lips and fingers. As a lotion it is commonly mixed with Calendula, Homoeopaths call this lotion Hypercal.

Part Used - Aerial parts

Dose - 1 to 4mls of tincture 3 times a day. In the tea form 3 to 4 cups per day.

Peppermint

Actions - Carminative, diaphoretic, anti-spasmodic, anti-emetic, nervine, analgesic, anti-septic.

Uses- Nausea, heartburn, indigestion, colic, flatulence, dyspepsia, vomiting, fevers, migraine headaches and irritable bowel syndrome (IBS).

Part Used - Leaf.

Dose - 1 to 2mls of tincture 3 times a day. In the tea form 3 to 4 cups per day.

Caution - May reduce milk flow if breast feeding.

Rescue Remedy

For First Aid use, emergencies and associated stress, use for any type of shock physical or emotional. Emotionally it will relieve that uptight feeling or apprehension before a certain event.

Rescue Remedy is a mixture of five Bach Flower Remedies and has been used since the late 30s so it has been well proved.

Dose - 4 drops in a little water and sipped.

Slippery Elm Bark Powder

Actions - Demulcent, emollient, nutrient, astringent. Slippery elm bark provides a nutritious gruel which also possesses remarkable medicinal properties acting as a poultice both internally and externally. A nutrient and food for very old or young or weak, coats and heals all inflamed tissues internally and externally and is used for the stomach, intestines, ulcers, ulcerative colitis, enteritis, dysentery, constipation and internal bleeding of the digestive tract.

Uses - Treatment of all digestive complaints especially ulcers for which it is a specific, dysentery, all pectoral disorders including TB, lung and bronchial hemorrhage, wasting diseases, rickets, stunted growth.

Externally - A poultice for all skin ailments especially old ailments and hard swellings.

Part Used - Inner Bark.

Dose - 1 part powder to 8 parts water.

Tea Tree Oil

Australian Tea Tree Oil is one of the world's best antiseptics and is also anti-bacterial, anti-fungal and anti-viral which means you can use it with good results on virtually any wound on the skin. The oil is good for drawing out infections, once they have been drawn out use Calendula to finish the healing.

Witch Hazel

Actions - Astringent one of the most widely used ones. Anti-septic.

As with all astringents this herb may be used wherever there is bleeding both externally and internally, commonly used for piles, bruises and inflamed swellings, varicose veins, diarrhea.

Uses - Internally to heal ulcerated and burnt tissues in cases of poisoning, stomach and intestinal ulcers, Externally - wounds, sores, bruises, ulcers, sore eyes and inflamed ears.

Part Used - Bark or leaves

Dose - Used mainly as a lotion 1 to 10 or as a cream.

Glossary Of Herbal Terms

Anti-microbial - Helps the body destroy or resist pathogenic micro-organisms.
Herbs - Aniseed, Cayenne, Calendula, Echinacea, Garlic, Peppermint, Rosemary, Sage, Thyme, Wormwood.

Antispasmodic - Prevents or eases spasms and cramps.
Herbs - Aniseed, Chamomile, Fennel, Lemon Balm, Passion Flower, Rosemary, Sage, Skullcap, St Johns Wort, Thyme, Valerian.

Astringent - Contracts tissue which in turn reduces discharges, these herbs contain tannins and usually have a antibacterial action.
Herbs - Agrimony, Calendula, Chickweed, Comfrey, Eyebright, Raspberry, Sage, Rosemary, St Johns Wort, Slippery Elm, Thyme, Witch Hazel.

Carminative - Stimulates peristalsis of the digestive system and relaxes the stomach and helps remove gas and wind from the system.
Herbs - Aniseed, Chamomile, Fennel, Garlic, Ginger, Lemon Balm, Parsley, Peppermint, Sage, Rosemary, Thyme, Valerian.

Demulcent - Soothes and protects irritated or inflamed internal tissues.
Herbs - Corn Silk, Comfrey, Fenugreek, Licorice, Marshmallow, Oats, Plantain, Slippery Elm.

Diaphoretic - Aids the skin in the elimination of toxins and produces sweat.
Herbs - Chamomile, Fennel, Garlic, Ginger, Lemon Balm, Peppermint, Sarsaparilla, Thyme.

Emetic - Causes vomiting.

Emollient - Acts externally the way demulcents do internally.
Herbs - Chickweed, Comfrey, Fenugreek, Slippery Elm.

Infusion - Is like how you make a cup of tea but when you make herb teas you don't use milk. The teas you will be making here are mainly Peppermint and Chamomile tea. Pour boiling water onto the tea bag in the cup and cover the cup (to stop the essential oils from evaporating) and leave for about 5 minutes. To sweeten add honey.

Lotion - A water and tincture mixture example 2 parts tincture to 20 parts water.

Nervine - Has a beneficial effect on the nervous system.
Herbs - Chamomile, Oats, Peppermint, Rosemary, Skullcap, St Johns Wort, Thyme, Valerian.

Tincture - Herbal tinctures are made from herbs mixed with a water and alcohol mix of about half and half and are usually of the strength of 1 part herb to 5 parts solvent.

Notes

Homoeopathy

Homoeopathy is one of the hardest of the Natural Therapies to master and requires a lot of work and effort to do the job as it is meant to be done. The main principle and rule is that like cures like. So you have to match the symptoms of the <u>dis - ease </u>with the known symptoms that a remedy causes. The closer the match with the known symptoms of a disorder with those of the remedy the higher the Potency (strength) you use. With this First Aid Kit I am using all the remedies in a Low Potency mainly the 6C Potency because I know they will generally cover most of the symptoms but will not be exact all the time. So instead of using the remedies like a sniper concentrating on exactness we will be using them in the shot gun approach, in other words we are aiming to hit a very wide and broad area. This book is meant as a introduction into Homoeopathy and in using it you shall learn that it works and is very effective and once you have proven its worth to yourself you may wish to study it further. Homoeopathy is a very complex science and I could go for pages and pages in just explaining how it works but I feel that the best way for you to learn is to try it for yourself and take it from there. Read the list of remedies below and become familiar with what they can do and what they treat and above all always follow the normal First Aid procedures and use your common sense and you shouldn't have many problems.

A Warning About Potencies And Handling Homoeopathic Remedies.

1. Remedies should be touched as little as possible as the heat and moisture of your hands can spoil them.

2. Do not transfer remedies from one container to another as the potencies are easily contaminated by another remedy.

3. Keep potencies away from strong smelling products such as perfume, soap, incense, essential oils, peppermints, coffee and anything containing peppermint or menthol. Menthol is used in homoeopathy to antidote any remedies that is giving a bad reaction.

4. Keep away from heat and light; try to keep them under 40 degrees Celsius.

Taking The Potencies

1. Dissolve under the tongue.

2. Do not swallow with a drink; the potencies are absorbed through the membranes in the mouth.

3. Do not eat, drink, smoke or clean teeth for about 15 minutes before or after taking a remedy.

Dosage For The Potencies

1. For minor problems take one twice daily up to 7 to 10 days.

2. For acute problems take one every 2 to 4 hours up till 2 days. Reduce to 3 times daily for a further 3 to 5 days.

3. For very serious problems one every 5 to 15

minutes for 6 to 8 doses or until relief is obtained.

Homoeopathic First Aid Remedies

Aconite

Aconite is best used in the first stages of a illness, especially when fear and anxiety are present.

Symptoms appear suddenly, without warning and they may be caused by exposure to cold winds or draughts or by a severe fright. Symptoms are a marked restlessness, extreme anxiety or fear, high fever with a burning skin, extreme sweating and a burning thirst, a hoarse dry painful cough, bright light noises stress and cold worsen the symptoms, rest and quiet relieves the symptoms. The pains of Acconite are unbearable, sharp, shooting, burning pains, tingling and numbness.

Allium Cepa

Characteristic symptoms of this remedy are increased secretions from the eyes and nose, like those of the common cold. Frequent sneezing with watery discharge which burns the nose and upper lip, but the eye discharge is bland and doesn't burn (the opposite of Euphrasia). Tickling in the throat with incessant cough (feels as if larynx is split) holds throat when coughing. Being in cool open air relieves the symptoms.

Apis

Apis is used for various types of swelling and inflammation such as that from animal bites and bites and stings from insects; it is also used for measles, mumps, sore throats, sore red eyes and fever. Apis is a quick acting remedy for inflammations especially those ones with edema and lots of swelling which is its main use. Symptoms are swelling with edema which makes the effected parts look shiny, red and puffy, the swollen parts feel soggy and waterlogged, a fever that develops rapidly but without thirst, extreme restlessness and fidgeting, an irritable nature and perhaps jealous, cool air and cold compresses relieve the symptoms. Pains are burning and stinging.

Arnica

Bruises and similar injuries where the skin is unbroken and there is mental or emotional shock. Symptoms are any type of bruising or similar injury caused by crushing, squeezing or wrenching, muscles strains which feel sore and bruised, shock after accidents, there is a fear of being touched because of the pain, good for the soreness after birth and medical operations.

The kit contains Arnica in potency and also as a cream. The cream must not be used on broken skin or wounds.

Bellis Perennis

Trauma to abdomen and pelvic organs especially after surgery and child birth if Arnica does not give relief. Injuries to the nerves with intense soreness, back ache from hard physical work such as gardening, pain is bruised sore and aching, better cold presses, worse touch, after getting wet.

Calendula

We use this in the tincture form and make lotions from the tincture. The part used is the Flowers and it is used for wounds and skin irritations, it is healing, soothing, anti-inflammatory, astringent, anti-fungal and anti-microbial.

Use For - Cuts, grazes, infected sores, fungal infections, any skin inflammations, regulates the oil production of the skin so is good for acne, to stop bleeding, for bruises and sprains, skin ulcers and minor burns and scolds.

Cantharis

Important first aid remedy for minor burns and for other pains that feel burning and fiery, also has a healing effect on the bladder, urethra and other parts of the urinary tract where burning pain is the key symptom., burns and scalds especially where blistering and inflammation occur, sunburn, insect bites that feel hot and burn, cystitis. Pains are violent burning, cutting, stabbing or smarting, rawness.

Better from warmth rest and rubbing.

Causticum

Burns and burning pains such as cystitis also used for coughs, burns to the skin especially with marked inflammation and blistering, coughs, laryngitis and hoarseness from straining and over using voice, cystitis especially with involuntary passing of urine when coughing, exposure to cold dry air may make symptoms worse.

Euphrasia

Affects the mucous membranes of the eyes, nose and chest producing copious watery secretions, eye secretions cause smarting of the skin while the nose discharge is bland. used for conjunctivitis, eye strain generally but especially from computers, eyes that feel sore and inflamed and look red, hay fever symptoms including a tickly throat, sneezing, a runny nose, and itchy red watering eyes. Sunlight wind and warmth worsen the symptoms.

Hypericum

Used for bruises and other injuries especially to nerve rich areas like the fingers, lips, ears, eyes ,tail bone, good for the pain of puncture wounds of any cause eg animal or insect. Helps with the pains after operations especially amputations. Pains are violent shooting pains along a nerve path, burning, tingling and numbness. Worse from shock and touch and better from rubbing

Ledum

Has a action on the capillaries and is useful for cleaning up bruises especially around the eyes, mainly used for puncture wounds made by sharp points such as nails and wood splinters and insect bites and stings especially ones that don't heal properly and look purple and puffy. Wounds that feel cold to the touch, septic conditions, sprains, pains are throbbing, tearing ,prickling, they shoot upwards, stiff and sore. Better cold, cold bathing.

Ruta

Has effects on the joints, tendons, cartilages, and the periosteum which is a fine membrane that covers bones and gives the shiny look it is also used for eye strain where the vision goes dim. Used for painful bruises affecting the bones, strains to the tendons or joints, aching with restlessness, pains are gnawing, digging, burning, bruised, sore as if beaten, banes as if broken, pain deep in the bones. Worse from over exertion, touch, cold wet weather. Better from lying and warmth.

Rescue Remedy

Is one of the Bach Flower remedies or to be more exact is a mixture of four Bach Flower remedies.

Rescue remedy is used for shock of any kind physical or emotional and has been well proven to be effective over the years.

Staphysagria

Suits sensitive people who suppress their feelings and suffer in silence or who boil over with indignation, remedy for cut and wounds especially those that are from medical procedures and have the mentioned feelings. The pains are stinging, stitching, smarting, squeezing, as if stabbed by a knife. Worse from touch, emotions and suppressed anger.

Symphytum

Causes bone to grow and promotes fast healing. Used for injuries to the hard parts of the body while Arnica is for the soft parts. Also used for eye injuries caused from blows.

Caution - do not use if a pin has been placed in the bone as the pin has to be removed latter.

Tarentula Cubensis

For abscesses, boils, carbuncles, swellings of any kind but especially on the back of the neck where the skin turns black, red/blue or purple. with great pain. Deep septic conditions with hardening of the effected part, condition comes on fast, pains are burning, stinging, throbbing, pricking like a needle.

www.ingramcontent.com/pod-product-compliance
Lightning Source LLC
Chambersburg PA
CBHW051237170526
45165CB00004B/1469